# Gluten Free

## *Your Complete Guide To The Healthiest Gluten Free Foods Along With Delicious & Energizing Gluten Free Cooking Recipes*

By Ace McCloud
Copyright © 2014

# Disclaimer

The information provided in this book is designed to provide helpful information on the subjects discussed. This book is not meant to be used, nor should it be used, to diagnose or treat any medical condition. For diagnosis or treatment of any medical problem, consult your own physician. The publisher and author are not responsible for any specific health or allergy needs that may require medical supervision and are not liable for any damages or negative consequences from any treatment, action, application or preparation, to any person reading or following the information in this book. Any references included are provided for informational purposes only. Readers should be aware that any websites or links listed in this book may change.

# Table of Contents

Introduction ............................................................. 5
Chapter 1: What Gluten Is & Foods That Contain Gluten..... 7
Chapter 2: Gluten-Free Foods .............................. 10
Chapter 3: Delicious Gluten-Free Breakfasts .................... 13
Chapter 4: Tasty Gluten-Free Lunch Recipes .................... 19
Chapter 5: Healthy Gluten-Free Snacking ........................ 27
Chapter 6: Easy To Prepare Gluten-Free Dinners ............. 31
Conclusion ............................................................. 39
My Other Books and Audio Books ........................................40

# Be sure to check out my website for all my Books and Audio books.
## www.AcesEbooks.com

# Introduction

I want to thank you and congratulate you for buying the book, "Gluten Free: Your Complete Guide To The Healthiest Gluten Free Foods Along With Delicious & Energizing Gluten Free Recipes."

If there is one thing that everyone likes to do, it's to eat! The different foods that you eat provide your body with important vitamins and minerals that help keep you healthy and energized throughout the day. Most people commonly eat breakfast, lunch and dinner with some snacks in between. While it is important to watch your weight as well as what you're putting in your body, it is easy for most people to eat whatever they want. With the abundance of different grocery stores, restaurants and farm markets as well as food companies and manufacturers, many kinds of ingredients go into most foods today.

Many people have been curious about a gluten-free diet due to a recent health trend where lots of celebrities and professionals have been promoting their surge in wellbeing after eliminating gluten from their diet. A gluten-free diet generally avoids foods that contain wheat, rye and barley as well as other foods and additives that have ingredients that contain these substances. While most peoples' bodies are able to withstand most foods and ingredients, not everybody's can. Even if you do not suffer from Celiac disease, gluten can leave you feeling drained and lethargic. Celiac disease is an autoimmune disorder that prompts your body to attack itself rather than an allergy. This disease specifically targets the upper third portion of the small intestine. Right now, experts believe that the best method for treatment of Celiac disease is to follow a diet that is gluten-free. The word gluten describes certain types of storage proteins that are found in different types of grains, commonly wheat, rye and barley. If you have Celiac disease and you maintain a diet that consists of those substances, your body will in turn begin to damage your small intestine. Once your small intestine begins to get damaged, your body will have a more difficult time absorbing the nutrients found in food and you can in turn become malnourished and weak.

The good news is that a gluten-free diet can benefit everyone, not just people who suffer from Celiac disease. The biggest benefit of following a gluten-free diet is that your body and mind can feel much better overall. Following a gluten-free diet can alleviate fatigue, headaches, joint pain, mood disorders, gastrointestinal problems, insomnia, neurological problems, seizures, respiratory problems, lactose intolerance, skin disorders, weight problems and autoimmune disorders. This is in part due to the fact that a gluten-free diet does not contain overly processed foods and focuses more on fruits, vegetables and other all-natural foods.

In this book you will discover the best recipes and cooking instructions for preparing delicious gluten-free meals for any time of the day. Most of these recipes will take you less than 30 minutes to prepare and the end results are amazing! After following some of the recipes and tips in this book, you will be able to eat like a king, regardless of whether or not your body has gluten intolerance. Be prepared to say goodbye to lethargy and hello to a super energized and healthy life!

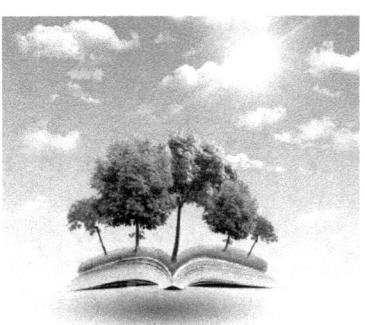

# Chapter 1: What Gluten Is & Foods That Contain Gluten

One of the most obvious signs that may point to gluten intolerance is if you have specific digestive issues such as constipation, diarrhea, bloating and/or gas. After you eat a meal that contains high gluten content, you may feel tired or have an unclear mind. You may also experience neurological symptoms, such as feeling dizzy or nausea. Another common sign of gluten intolerance is migraine headaches along with hormone imbalances, joint pain and inflammation along with mood swings.

Celiac disease can be tiring and painful. Doctors have found that some people even experience recurring symptoms, many of which include constipation and obesity. Celiac disease can also bring on other side effects such as anemia, osteoporosis, dermatitis, dental problems, nerve damage, joint pain and acid reflux. While the cause of this disease is currently unknown, doctors estimate that about 1 in 141 people will develop this disease. Often times, it goes undiagnosed.

While you should always consult your doctor for an official diagnosis, eating a gluten-free diet can still benefit most people, as it mostly focuses on "natural" foods such as fruits, vegetables, meats, fish, etc. For a quick video that explains Gluten very nicely, be sure to check out the YouTube video Gluten by SciShow.

Regardless of whether they suffer from Celiac disease, some people believe in eating a gluten-free diet anyway. The best way to know for sure if you are suffering from Celiac disease or intolerance is to contact your doctor. He or she can give you some tests, ask you questions, and work with you to figure out if you need to follow a gluten-free diet or just reduce the amount of Gluten you are currently eating.

I have personally started reducing the gluten in my diet about a month before the publishing of this book and have noticed a nice difference in my energy levels and mental clarity. I haven't totally eliminated it from my diet, but I have made a bunch of simple and healthier dietary changes that has reduced my consumption of gluten by a lot. Some of the changes I made was a lot more fruits and vegetables in my diet, I stopped eating bread and crackers, a bit more meat, along with several other diet choices that are healthy with low or no gluten content. Everyone is different. Be sure to try reducing the gluten in your diet for a month, keeping a food journal and just see how you feel afterwards. Many people will notice a lot of positive benefits if this is done the right way. Be sure to check out all the recipes in the following chapters that will make the process fun and energy packed!

**Foods That Contain Gluten**

If you suffer from Celiac disease or if you're just trying to go gluten-free for better health, the first and most important thing that you need to know is how to maintain a proper diet. Below is a list of the majority of foods that generally contain gluten:

- Pasta
- Breads
- Couscous
- Muffins
- Cookies
- Bouillon cubes
- Cakes
- Croutons
- Breadcrumbs
- Flour Tortillas
- Crackers
- Soup broth
- Cereals
- Pastries
- Gravy
- Oats
- Beer
- Certain candies
- Fried food
- Most sauces
- Most dressings
- Hot dogs
- Lunch meats
- Fried fish
- Matzo
- Modified food starch
- Malt
- Seasoned snacks
- Soysauce

In general, most grains such as wheat, barley, rye, white flour, whole wheat, white flour, semolina, wheat germ, wheat bran, and other wheat-based flours contain gluten. You should also avoid kamut, triticale, durum wheat, graham flour, and spelt. Experts in gluten-free diets also advise to avoid commercially processed oats, although pure oats are generally safe. As always, the best way to ensure that a good is safe for a gluten-free diet is to read the label of the food you are purchasing.

When going grocery shopping, it is important to keep some things in mind. If you plan on buying lunch meats, it is a good idea to buy the prepackaged kind.

Freshly sliced lunch meats are good but there is more of a risk for contamination if the slicer is not properly cleaned in between cuts. If you are really against prepackaged lunch meats, you should always ask the deli employees to fully clean and sanitize the slicer before cutting your meats. Also try to avoid buying anything that is thrown together in a bin or box. When foods are mixed together like that, there is more of a risk of cross-contamination. Always go for the foods that are neatly placed on the shelves.

Look out for specific gluten-free brands on the shelves. These brands are often gluten-free alternatives to foods that you would normally enjoy. Some of the best known gluten-free brands in most grocery stores in the USA are Glutino, Udi's Gluten Free Foods, Ancient Harvest, Blue Diamond Growers, Barlean's, Earthbound Farm, Applegate, Live G Free, and Nature's Path among more. Some bloggers on the website Stockpiling Moms have even come forward to put a complete list of gluten-free brands together.

Always look for the words "gluten-free" on the labels. The FDA has only made this a voluntary rule for now and any food that contains less than 20 parts per million (ppm) of gluten. Although this does not ensure that a product is 100% gluten-free, most experts believe that this would not be enough to trigger a reaction.

Check out this YouTube video, Gluten-Free Shopping With NFCA by the National Foundation for Celiac Awareness, to see what it's like to shop for gluten-free items. You can see some of the more popular gluten-free brands as well as get some good tips and ideas.

**What's Being Done About Celiac Disease?**

Currently, the University of Chicago is doing the most research on this disease. This school is working to raise awareness of the disease as well as work with diagnosis rates and training doctors. The non-profit organization that runs this program has assisted many people over the last couple of years with this disease and relies solely on donations to thrive. In the meantime, the best way that you can get to great health is to follow the right diet, which you will discover some great recipes for in the next few chapters!

# Chapter 2: Gluten-Free Foods

Now that you know which foods to avoid when you are following a gluten-free diet, it is time to discover which foods that you *can* eat. Below is a list of foods and ingredients that are gluten-free and safe to eat:

**Foods**

- Corn
- Rice
- Milk
- Butter
- Plain yogurt
- Fresh vegetables
- Cheese
- Fresh fruits
- Canola oil
- Seafood
- Meats
- Nuts, beans, legumes
- Eggs
- Distilled vinegar
- Spices

**Ingredients**

- Amaranth
- Annatto
- Buckwheat
- Glucose syrup
- Montina
- Millet
- Lecithin
- Quinoa
- Oat gum
- Teff
- Silicon dioxide
- Sorghum
- Lactose
- Soy
- Arrowroot
- Cornstarch
- Tapioca starch or flour
- Potato starch

- Vanilla

**Where to Buy Gluten-Free Foods**

You can buy most of the basic foods (like fruits, vegetables, meats, seafood, etc) at your local grocery store. However, many stores also carry more specific foods (like breads, cookies, pastas, etc.) as a gluten-free brand. Chapter One contains a link to some of the most popular brands of gluten-free foods. Alternatively, you can buy specific gluten-free foods online to make the hunt easier.

**Breakfasts**

Bisquick Pancake and Baking Mix, Gluten-Free

Right Foods Organic Oatmeal Cups

King Arthur Multipurpose Gluten-Free Flour

Whenever Bars

Udi's Gluten-Free Vanilla Granola

**Lunch/Dinner**

Annie's Homegrown Rice Pasta and Cheddar Mac and Cheese

Barilla Gluten-Free Spaghetti

Sam Mills Cheesy Burger

Hodgson Mill Gluten-Free Bread Mix

Stonewall Kitchen Herbed Pizza Crust Mix

**Snacks**

Glutino Gluten-Free Pretzel Sticks

Enjoy Life Soft Baked Cookies

Arrowhead Mills Gluten-Free Chocolate Cake Mix

Crunchmaster Multigrain Gluten-Free Crackers

Stonewall Kitchen Cinnamon Doughnut Mix

Additionally, you can buy most gluten-free brands in stores in the USA such as Walmart, Whole Foods Market, Trader Joe's, Aldi, Kroger, Shoprite, Stop and

Shop and Wegman's. From here on in, you will discover some of the best gluten-free recipes!

*Always check the label and packaging on any ingredient that you buy to ensure that it is gluten-free or low in gluten.*

One more quick note—in this book, I use the terms "small spoon" and "large spoon", which translate to "teaspoon" and "tablespoon" respectively.

# Chapter 3: Delicious Gluten-Free Breakfasts

You should always make time to eat breakfast because it starts you off with plenty of energy. It should never be skipped if you are trying to live your day at <u>peak performance</u>. This chapter will list some of the best and easiest to make gluten-free breakfasts that you can prepare for yourself or your family.

**Eggs with Salmon**

You will need:

- Six eggs
- Six ounces of salmon
- One large spoon of Old Bay seasoning
- Three large spoons of olive oil
- One diced onion
- Three large spoons of gluten-free flour
- One can of chicken broth
- One and a half cups of milk
- A dash of salt
- A dash of pepper
- One can of small peas
- Six English muffins, gluten-free

Put each egg in a large pan and pour in an inch of water. Allow to boil and then take out the eggs, allowing them to sit aside for 10 minutes. Put the eggs in cold water to easily peel and then cut them up. In another pan, put the salmon in with another cup of water and the seasoning. Allow to boil and then reduce heat and simmer. In a separate pan, heat up the olive oil and cook the onions for five minutes. Add in the flour and then mix together. Then add in the milk, salt, broth and pepper and cook for two minutes. Throw in the peas and allow them to cook for half a minute. Add the salmon and eggs to this mixture and then put it over the English muffins before serving.

**Homemade Trail Mix**

You will need:

- Two large handfuls of almonds, sliced
- One large handful of coconut flakes, unsweetened
- One large handful of macadamia nuts
- One large handful of pumpkin seeds
- One smaller handful of dried pineapple
- One smaller handful of dried mango
- One smaller handful of dried strawberries

Over medium heat, put the coconut flakes and almonds in a pan. Stir together until both come out toasted. Combine with the rest of the ingredients and divide up in small bags.

**Coconut Pancakes**

You will need:

- Two cups of brown rice flour
- One cup of corn starch
- Two small spoons of baking powder
- A dash of salt
- Two eggs
- Three small spoons of coconut oil, melted
- Three large spoons of coconut palm sugar
- One and a half cups of coconut milk
- Vanilla
- A handful of coconut flakes

Combine the flour, baking soda, salt and starch together. Add in the eggs, milk, oil, sugar and vanilla and whisk together. Slowly add in the flakes. Over medium heat, melt some more oil and slowly pour in the batter to make pancakes of your desired size. Cook for about five minutes on each side. To make syrup that goes with it, combine another cup of coconut palm sugar with half a cup of water and bring it to a boil. Simmer for 10 minutes and then stir in vanilla. Top off pancakes with syrup and more coconut flakes.

**Corned Beef Hash**

You will need:

- Six large peeled and diced potatoes
- One chopped onion
- One cup of beef broth
- One can of corned beef

Cut the corned beef into chunks. Then heat a skillet over a medium flame and add in the corned beef, potatoes, beef broth and onions. Cover the skillet and let simmer until all of the liquid has dissolved. Toss together and serve.

**Gluten-Free Banana Bread**

You will need:

- 5 mashed, extra ripe bananas

- One third cup of melted butter
- One third cup of all natural maple syrup
- One third cup of coconut flour
- One and a half cups of millet flower
- Two small spoons of baking power
- Three small spoons of vanilla extract
- Two small spoons of cinnamon
- Two eggs

Preheat your oven and grease a loaf pan. Mix together the bananas, melted butter, maple syrup, eggs, and vanilla extract. In a separate, smaller bowl, mix together the coconut flour, millet flour, baking powder, and cinnamon. Pour the smaller bowl into the larger bowl and mix together until smooth. Pour the batter into the pan and bake for 45 minutes. Let it sit for a while before serving.

**Gluten-Free Pancakes**

You will need:

- 124 grams of gluten-free white flour
- 250 ml of milk
- One egg
- A bit of butter to fry them in

Combine the flour, one quarter of milk, and egg in a bowl and whisk together until it is pasty. Then add in some more milk and mix well. Add in the remaining milk and wait for 20 minutes. Stir one more time before you get ready to use it. In a pan, melt some butter and then slowly pour the mixture in until you form pancakes. Fry each side until it is light brown and continue to do so until you have as many pancakes as you want. You can optionally top off each pancake with agave syrup.

**Gluten-Free Quinoa Porridge**

You will need:

- One half cup of quinoa flakes
- One cup of unsweetened almond milk
- Four dried prunes, chopped
- Half a large spoon of sliced almonds
- One large spoon of vanilla extract
- One small spoon of ginger
- One pinch of cinnamon
- An eighth of a small spoon of nutmeg

Boil the almond milk in a pot and add the quinoa flakes. Cook for 30 seconds while constantly stirring. Add the nutmeg, ginger, vanilla, cinnamon, and prunes and cook for an additional 30 seconds. Take the mixture off the heat, let it cool, and add the maple syrup while mixing it. Top it off the sliced almonds and serve.

**Gluten-Free Fruit Parfait**

You will need:

- 300g of rolled oats, gluten-free
- 180g of a mixture of nuts and seeds
- 180grams of dried fruit
- 125ml of apple juice
- A small amount of cinnamon
- One large spoon of vanilla extract
- One large helping of all natural maple syrup
- 60ml of coconut oil
- One small spoon of sea salt
- One quarter small spoon of black pepper

Preheat your oven to 325 degrees and combine the nuts and seeds, dried fruit, and oats into a big bowl. In a saucepan, combine the salt, pepper, vanilla extract, cinnamon, maple syrup, apple juice, and coconut oil. Heat this mixture until the coconut oil turns into a liquid. Once you have this liquid, toss it to coat over the dry mixture. Bake the final mixture 45 minutes. Let sit for a while after baking to get harder. Once the granola is made, you can serve it over yogurt.

**Gluten-Free Berry Muffins**

You will need:

- Two cups of raspberries or other berry of your choice
- Half a cup of water
- 2.5 cups of organic almond flour
- Two small spoons of cinnamon
- Half a small spoon of baking soda
- 3 large spoons of flaxseed
- Half a small spoon of vanilalla extract
- One quarter cup of agave syrup
- Three eggs
- Two large spoons of melted coconut oil

Preheat your oven to 350 degrees combine all of the dry ingredients together in a bowl. In a different bowl, combine all of the wet ingredients, adding the coconut oil last. Combine the wet and dry ingredients while also adding the berries. Line a muffin tray with cupcake holders and pour the batter into each hole. Bake for about 30 minutes and serve.

**Gluten-Free Banana Nut Bars**

You will need:

- Three mashed bananas
- Raw vanilla protein powder, two scoops
- One quarter cup of sliced almonds
- Two large spoons of raw coconut powder
- One small spoon of vanilla
- A small amount of cinnamon
- One large spoon of water
- A small amount of sweetener

Mix all ingredients into a bowl until there are no lumps. Line a cookie sheet with paper and smooth out. Store in refrigerator for 30 minutes and cut into pieces. Keep pieces refrigerated to stay fresh.

**Strawberry Coconut Smoothie**

You will need:

- One cup of fresh strawberries
- One frozen banana
- 3/4 cup of canned coconut milk
- One large spoon of chia seeds
- Half a cup of water
- One small spoon of vanilla extract

Combine all ingredients in a blender and blend until smooth. Top off with shredded cocounut for an added coconut flavor.

**Banana Pecan Waffles**

You will need:

- Four mashed bananas
- Two cups of unsweetened vanilla almond milk, room temperature
- Two thirds cup of melted coconut oil
- 13 drops of liquid sweetener
- A small amount of vanilla
- Two cups of gluten free flour
- One small spoon of baking powder

- One dash of sea salt
- One small spoon of ground nutmeg
- One large handful of unsalted, chopped pecans

Turn on your waffle iron and let it heat up. Be sure to grease it with some non-stick cooking spray. In a bowl, combine the mashed banana, coconut oil, and unsweetened almond milk. Also add the liquid sweetener and vanilla extract. Next, add in the flour, nutmeg, salt and baking powder. Stir the mixture well, add in the pecans, and let sit for 5 minutes. Afterwards, put one cup of the batter on the waffle iron and cook for about 5 minutes. Top off with one sliced banana, more pecans, and some all-natural maple syrup.

**Gluten-free Eggs in Tomato Shells**

You will need:

- One tomato
- One egg
- One large spoon of grated parmesean cheese
- One large spoon of minced chives
- Salt and pepper

Preheat your oven and grease a glass dish. Cut the top portion of the tomato off and empty the insides. Salt and pepper the inside and then turn it upside down to fully drain. Crack open the egg into the tomato inside and bake it for 20 minutes. Top with chives and cheese and melt in the warm oven.

**Blueberry Oatmeal Smoothie**

You will need:

- One half a cup of gluten free rolled oats
- One cup of soy milk
- One frozen banana
- Three quarter cup of organic blueberries
- One large spoon of honey
- Five ice cubes (only if using fresh berries)

First blend the oats in a blender until they get grounded down. Next, add the rest of the ingredients, blend again, and then serve.

# Chapter 4: Tasty Gluten-Free Lunch Recipes

Lunch is another important meal of the day. It is meant to give your body an early morning/afternoon boost once you've burned off all the energy you've gotten from your breakfast. This chapter provides some really delicious, easy and simple gluten-free lunch recipes to keep you going before dinner.

**Vegetable Pasta**

You will need:

- Eight ounces of gluten-free fettuccine made with brown rice
- A dash of salt
- Half a cup of olive oil
- Black pepper
- Two bell peppers
- Two corn ears
- Two zucchinis
- A pint of grape tomatoes, halved
- One cup of basil leaves
- Four ounces of goat cheese

Add salt to water in a pot and bring it to a boil. Cook the pasta and put one cup of the water aside. Drain the pasta and put it back in the pan. Over medium heat, cut and grill up all the vegetables, turning each one frequently. Add the grilled vegetables to the pasta and add in the half of the water. Toss with the basil and goat cheese.

**Spinach Omelet**

You will need:

- Two eggs
- One bag of fresh spinach leaves
- Two large spoons of grated Parmesan
- A dash of onion powder
- A dash of nutmeg
- Salt
- Pepper

Beat the eggs and in add in the Parmesan and spinach. Add in all the spices. Coat a skillet with cooking spray over medium heat and cook the mixture for three minutes. Using a spatula, flip it and cook it for another 3 minutes. Next, simmer for 3 more minutes then serve.

## Apple Smoothie

You will need:

- One cup of almond milk, unsweetened
- One cup of applesauce, unsweetened
- Half a cup of unsalted, water-soaked cashews
- Two small spoons of vanilla
- Half a small spoon of ground cinnamon
- Two large spoons of all natural maple syrup
- One cup of ice

Mix all ingredients together in your blender until they come out smooth and consistent, usually blending for about one minute.

## Black Beans With Rice

You will need:

- One large spoon of vegetable oil
- One small spoon of dried oregano
- One small spoon of garlic powder
- One chopped onion
- One can of un-drained black beans
- One can of stewed tomatoes
- Two cups of instant brown rice, uncooked

Heat oil in a large skillet over medium heat. Add in the onion and cook until it softens. Next add the beans, oregano, garlic powder, and tomatoes. Boil the mixture and then add in the rice. Cover the skillet and simmer for five minutes. Allow it to cool off before serving.

## Apricot Flavored Chicken

You will need:

- Two pounds of chopped and pitted apricots
- One small cup of sugar
- Two large spoons of cider vinegar
- Two pounds of cubed chicken breast
- Salt
- One large spoon of butter, unsalted
- Three large spoons of olive oil
- Chopped onion
- Two cans of chicken broth

- One large spoon of rosemary, chopped
- A dash of cinnamon
- Two small spoons of hot sauce
- Pepper

Combine the apricots with the vinegar and sugar. Let that mixture sit for a while as you heat up the butter and one spoon of olive oil over medium heat. Cook all of the chicken breasts until they are well done and then cut into pieces. Salt the chicken as it browns. Put the rest of the olive oil in the skillet and cook the onion until it softens. Pour in the chicken broth and turn the heat to low. Take two-thirds of the apricots into a blender and puree. Pour that mixture into the chicken broth mixture. Next, add in the hot sauce, cinnamon and rosemary. Simmer the entire mixture for 20 minutes. Simmer the chicken and last half of the apricots for five minutes and then serve all together with rice.

**Gluten-Free Pizza**

You will need:

- One large spoon of yeast
- One and a third cup of milk
- One small spoon of sugar
- Two and one half cups of gluten-free flour
- Two large spoons of xanthan gum
- Salt
- Two large spoons of olive oil
- Two large spoons of cider vinegar
- One third cup of gluten-free corn meal

Preheat your oven to 400 degrees and mix the yeast and sugar with warmed up milk. Next, add in the flour, gum and salt. You'll know if you're doing it right if the mixture is foaming. After that, add in the oil and cider vinegar, followed by the flour. Mix all ingredients together. Add some flour to a piece of parchment paper and roll out the dough, topping it with the corn meal. Make the dough thin like a pizza and then bake it until it turns golden. Once the dough is formed, you can top it off with whatever you want—usually cheese, sauce, and some healthy toppings. Melt the new toppings by warming up in the oven.

**Asian Lettuce Wraps**

You will need:

- One serving of lettuce leaves
- One large spoon of gluten-free soy sauce
- Two large spoons of gluten-free oyster sauce
- One large spoon of dry sherry

- One small spoon of sugar
- One large spoon of sesame oil
- One slice of minced ginger
- One minced garlic clove
- Two green onions, chopped
- One pound of chicken breasts
- One diced red pepper
- One can of water chestnuts
- One cup of diced celery
- One small spoon of corn starch paired with two large spoons of water

Prepare the lettuce by washing it and peeling the leaves apart. Next, mix together the soy sauce, oyster sauce, sherry and sugar. Put that mixture aside. Over high heat, add the sesame oil to a skillet and cook the ginger, garlic and green onions together until you can smell them. Add in the chicken and cook until the chicken is well done. Take the chicken out of the pan and then replace with the sauce and turn to medium heat. Also add in the corn starch and water. Stir everything together to make it thick. Put the chicken back in and cook for about three minutes. Flatten out the lettuce leaves and put some of the chicken and sauce into each one, folding it like a taco. Do this for all leaves and then serve.

## Arugula Salad

You will need:

- Peeled, boiled beets cut into strips
- Arugula
- A handful of goat cheese
- A handful of chopped walnuts
- One quarter cup of olive oil
- Half of a lemon
- One quarter small spoon of powdered mustard
- Three quarters of a small spoon of Sugar
- Salt and pepper

Toss together the beets, arugula, goat cheese and walnuts. For the dressing, mix together the olive oil, lemon, powdered mustard, and sugar. Top off with salt and pepper as you want and serve.

## Chicken and Bean Salad

You will need:

- A garlic clove
- One dash of salt

- Six large spoons of olive oil, extra virgin
- Six large spoons of OJ
- One quarter cup of wine vinegar
- One large spoon of Dijon
- One 15oz can of white beans
- Five cooked chicken breasts, diced
- Three diced zucchini
- One and a half cups of diced celery
- One quarter cup of feta cheese
- One cup of chopped basil leaves
- Two cups of torn romaine
- Two cups of radicchio leaves

Use the first list of ingredients to make the salad dressing. Peel and mash the garlic while adding it to one quarter small spoon of salt. Mix together in a small bowl to make a paste. Add the olive oil and whisk. Next, add the orange juice, mustard, and vinegar and blend together. Set aside while you prepare the salad. For the salad portion, put together the chicken, zucchini, beans, cheese, and celery and blend together. Add in the basil and some of the dressing and toss. In a medium bowl, toss the mixture with the romaine and radicchio and serve.

**Gluten-Free Greek Salad**

You will need:

- Three large spoons of lemon juice
- Two large spoons of olive oil, extra virgin
- One minced garlic clove
- Two small spoons of dried oregano
- One half small spoon of freshly ground pepper
- Three tomatoes
- One cucumber
- One can of chickpeas
- One third cup of feta cheese crumbles
- One quarter cup of red onion, thinly sliced
- Two large spoons of Kalamata olives, sliced
- Two cans of sardines

In a large bowl, combine the oil, garlic, lemon juice, pepper and oregano and whisk together. Cut the tomato and cucumber into chunks and add them in along with the onion, olives, feta, and chickpeas. Top off the salad with the sardines.

**Gluten-Free Roasted Pumpkin Soup with Apple**

You will need:

- Four pounds of pumpkin or butternut squash
- Four large sweet apples
- One quarter cup olive oil, extra virgin
- One and one quarter small spoons of salt
- One quarter small spoon of pepper
- One large spoon of chopped sage
- Six cups of chicken or vegetable broth
- One third cups of toasted hazelnuts
- Two large spoons of hazelnut oil

Preheat your oven to 450 degrees and toss the pumpkin or squash (peeled, cut and seeded) with the diced apples, olive oil, salt and pepper. Spread the mixture on a baking sheet and roast it for 30 minutes, stirring once. Add the sage and roast for another 15 minutes. Add one-third of the apples and pumpkin to a blender and add the broth. Blend together until smooth. Do this two more times for the remaining batches and heat it up over medium heat for 6 minutes, stirring occasionally. Top off each portion with the hazelnuts and hazelnut oil.

## Lentil and Rice Salad

You will need:

- Two large spoons of olive oil, extra virgin
- Two large spoons of red wine vinegar
- One large spoon shallot, finely chopped
- One large spoon mustard, Dijon
- One half small spoon of paprika
- One dash of salt
- One dash of pepper
- Two cups of brown rice, cooked
- One can of rinsed lentils
- One diced carrot
- Two large spoons of parsley, fresh and chopped

In a large bowl, blend together the vinegar, oil, mustard, shallot, paprika, salt and pepper. Once that is whisked together add in the lentils, rice, parsley and carrots. Stir it all together and serve. Refrigerate any left overs.

## Gluten-Free Chicken Tenders

You will need:

- Ten corn tortillas
- One quarter cup of gluten-free flour

- One cup of buttermilk
- Ten chicken tenders
- Two cups of vegetable oil
- A small cup of mustard
- A small cup of honey

Pulse the tortillas in a food processor until it looks coarse. Sprinkle in salt and pepper to season and then set aside. Coat the chicken tenders in the flour and then with the buttermilk and then roll in the tortilla mixture. On your stove top, heat some oil over a medium flame and cook the chicken tenders for about 6 minutes on each side. Drain on paper towels and combine the honey and mustard for a dipping sauce.

## Gluten-Free Macaroni and Cheese

You will need:

- Half a stick of butter
- One large handful of gluten-free puffed rice cereal
- One ounce of grated Parmesan
- One yellow onion, diced
- Two large spoons of potato starch
- Two cups of warm milk
- One bag of shredded cheddar cheese
- One small spoon of mustard, Dijon
- Salt and pepper

Preheat your oven and grease up a deep baking dish. Mix a small amount of the butter with the Parmesan and the puffed rice. In a separate, medium pan, melt the remainder of the butter. Cook the onion until it is soft and sprinkle in the potato starch, cooking for one minute. Slowly add the milk and whisk together until thick. Remove the mixture from the heat and add the cheddar and mustard. Add in the pasta and stir together. Top it off with the cereal mixture and bake for 20 minutes.

## Gluten-Free Spring Rolls

You will need:

- Three sheets of rice paper
- One large spoon of mayonnaise (reduced fat)
- One large spoon of sriracha
- One cup of shredded carrots
- One cup of chopped broccoli
- Two sliced bell peppers

- One cup of sliced mushrooms
- Six ounces of chicken breast, tofu, or turkey (your choice)

In a small bowl, mix together the mayonnaise and sriracha to make the dressing. Next, fill a dish with hot water and submerge each sheet of rice paper in it. Take it out of the water and lay on a towel. Spread the sauce on the paper and then add the vegetables and protein. Roll into the shape of an egg roll. Repeat this process for the other two rolls and enjoy.

**Gluten-Free Tuna Salad Sandwich**

You will need:

- One whole wheat French baguette (make sure it is gluten-free)
- One cup of thinly sliced red onion
- Half a cup of feta cheese
- One and one half cups of chopped cucumber
- Three sliced Roma tomatoes
- One dash of pepper
- One head of chopped red leaf lettuce
- Half a cup of tuna in water
- A small amount of white wine vinegar
- One small spoon of Dijon
- One large spoon of olive oil

Slice the baguette in half and remove most of the inside to create a shell. In a bowl, mix the tomatoes, onion, cucumber, and feta together. In another bowl, combine the mustard and vinegar while whisking in the olive oil. Pour this mixture over the vegetable mixture and top with the pepper. Add the lettuce leaves to the bottom half of the bread and then add the vegetable mixture. Next, add the tuna and replace the top half of the bread. Wrap in plastic for 10 minutes to allow the bread to absorb flavor and then serve.

# Chapter 5: Healthy Gluten-Free Snacking

In between lunch and dinner, it is easy to get hungry again. Snacking in between meals (healthily, of course) is a good way to keep energy flowing throughout your body all day and it helps hold you over until your last meal of the day. This chapter provides some easy and healthy gluten-free snacks that you will likely find yourself enjoying time after time.

## Cinnamon Apple Chips

You will need:

- Two big apples
- Two small spoons of cinnamon
- Half a small spoon of nutmeg
- One small spoon of sugar

Preheat your oven to 200 degrees and grease a baking sheet. Using a sharp knife cut each apple into thin slices. In a separate bowl, mix the cinnamon, nutmeg, and sugar and then cover each apple slice. Transfer the slices to the baking sheet and cook for about an hour and 45 minutes. Let cool before serving.

## Gluten-Free Sweet Potato French Fries

You will need:

- Two peeled sweet potatoes
- One large spoon of brown sugar
- Two large spoons of olive oil

Preheat your oven to 450 degrees and cut each sweet potato into french fry shapes. Put them on a baking sheet and cover with olive oil. Sprinkle on the brown sugar and salt/pepper if you prefer it. Bake on one side for 15 minutes and then bake on the other side for 10 minutes. Don't forget to eat them before they get too cold.

## Mint Chocolate Chip Shake

You will need:

- One frozen banana
- One large spoon of chocolate chips
- One quarter small spoon of peppermint extract
- One cup (more or less to thicken) of almond milk
- One quarter cup of frozen spinach

Simply blend all ingredients together in blender. You can add some flakes of chocolate to top it off.

**Toast with Avocado**

You will need:

- Half of an avocado
- One slice of toast, bread of your choice

Toast the bread and then spread the avocado the way you want. Some people like thick chunks of it on top and others may prefer a thinner layer. You can optionally add a slice of tomato to make it a more filling snack.

**Vegetable Smoothie**

You will need:

- One large handful of spinach leaves
- One cup of kale leaves, chopped
- One half of a pear
- One frozen banana
- Two servings of unsweetened almond milk
- One large spoon of honey

First, blend the milk, kale, and spinach together. Then add in the banana, honey, and pear. Blend together.

**Grain Free Crackers**

You will need:

- One cup of coconut flour
- One cup of almond flour
- One cup of arrowroot starch
- Two quarters cup of ground flax
- One cup of cashew milk
- One large spoon of sea salt
- One cup of coconut oil

Preheat your oven to 325 degrees and put a baking rack inside. In a food processor, blend together all ingredients using the pulse option. Do this until a dough forms. Shape the dough into a ball and thin it out using parchment paper. Thin it out like a cracker and try to make it consistent throughout. Take the top piece of paper away and place it on the baking rack. You can then start to cut your cracker shapes. Bake the dough for 20 minutes and let them cool. They will start to get crispy after they cool off.

**Raw Brownie Bits**

You will need:

- One cup of almonds
- One quarter cup of carob powder
- One quarter cup of raw honey
- One third cup of chia seeds
- Two large spoons of virgin coconut oil, cold-pressed
- One small spoon of vanilla extract
- One scoop of raw walnuts

Finely grind the almonds down in a food processor. Add in the carob powder and then grind it down again. Next, add the honey, chia seeds, coconut oil and vanilla and process together until mixed well. Roll the final product into "bites" and then store in the fridge for a few hours before serving

**Fried Plantains**

You will need:

- 4 green plantains
- A few spoons of coconut oil
- Salt

Peel the plantains and thinly slice them. Heat up the coconut oil in a pan and use it to fry up the plantains in a frying pan for about one minute each. Sprinkle a bit of salt on top and press the grease off them with a towel before serving.

**Quick Fix Gluten-Free Snacks**

- Sliced celery with almond butter
- Slice celery with cream cheese
- Slice apples with almond butter
- Dry assortments of fruit and rice
- Air-popped popcorn
- Hard boiled eggs
- Cottage cheese with melon
- Shrimp cocktail
- Raw vegetables with hummus for dipping
- Any type of fruit
- Cheese and fruit kabobs

**Ham and Cheese Bites**

You will need:

- One box of gluten-free bread mix
- Two large spoons of vegetable oil
- Three eggs
- One cup cheddar cheese, shredded
- One cup of diced ham
- Two large spoons of mustard
- One quarter cup of water
- A dash of salt
- One small spoon of dried onion

Preheat your oven to 375 degrees and prepare a baking sheet. Combine two eggs with the oil, bread mix, ham, cheese, water and mustard. When it forms into a dough, use your hands to make it smooth and consistent. Break off little pieces and roll them into bite sized shapes. Take the last egg and mix it with another small spoon of water. Spread that liquid over the dough along with the salt and dried onion. Let bake for fifteen minutes or until done.

# Chapter 6: Easy To Prepare Gluten-Free Dinners

Dinner is the last meal of the day, something that you often enjoy at home with your family after long hours of work. Dinner is often the most appetizing of meals and is something that many look forward too before settling in for the night. This chapter will provide some excellent, easy and healthy gluten-free dinner ideas that you can learn to prepare for yourself.

**Gluten-Free Stuffed Peppers**

You will need:
- One pound of ground beef
- Half a cup of brown rice
- One cup of water
- Six peppers (green)
- Two cans of tomato sauce
- One large spoon of gluten-free Worcestershire sauce
- A dash of garlic powder
- A dash of onion powder
- One small spoon of Italian seasoning
- Salt
- Pepper

Preheat your oven to 350 degrees and boil the rice. Once the water is boiling then simmer for 20 minutes. While you wait for the rice to simmer, cook the ground beef in a skillet until it is well done. Next, cut open the peppers on top and gut them. Place each hollowed out pepper facing upwards in an oven-safe dish. Combine the ground beef with the rice, one can of tomato sauce, onion powder, garlic powder, Worcestershire, salt and pepper. Add some of the mixture into the inside of each pepper. Add the Italian seasoning into the other can of tomato sauce and serve over the peppers. Bake for one hour and serve.

**Chicken Casserole with Rice**

You will need:

- Four pounds of chicken thighs, boneless
- Salt
- Pepper
- Olive oil
- One chopped onion
- Two minced cloves of garlic
- Half a pound of sliced button mushrooms
- One quarter cup of dry sherry

- One and one thirds cup of chicken broth
- Half a container of sour cream
- One quarter cup of cream
- One cup of white rice
- A dash salt
- One small spoon of Italian seasoning
- One small spoon of poultry seasoning
- A dash of paprika
- Two large spoons of parsley

Preheat your oven to 375 degrees. In a large pan, heat up some olive oil over medium heat and then add in a dash of salt. Cut the chicken thighs into smaller pieces and add to the pan, seasoning with more salt and pepper. Cook until each piece is browned, but not cooked all the way. Remove the chicken and add in some more olive oil. Cook the onions until they soften. Add in the garlic and cook for another minute or so. Transfer the onions and garlic to a casserole dish. Raise the heat a little and add in the mushrooms. Sauté and then transfer to the casserole dish. In the pan, add the dry sherry and then scrape off any brown bits on the surface. Next, turn the heat off and add in the chicken broth, cream, salt and sour cream. Stir together. After that, add the rice to the casserole dish and pour the cream mixture over it. Season with the paprika, Italian seasoning and poultry seasoning. Stir everything so that it is evenly distributed throughout the dish. Next, put the chicken on top of the rice mixture and wrap the top of the dish with aluminum foil. Bake for fifty minutes and then take out and remove the foil. If you find the casserole too runny, let it cook uncovered for a few more minutes. Top off with the parsley and then serve.

**Parmesan Chicken**

You will need:

- Six 6oz chicken breasts
- A dash of salt
- A dash of pepper
- Two large spoons of olive oil
- Three minced garlic cloves
- A handful of basil
- One lemon for juice
- One cup of gluten-free breadcrumbs
- Two thirds cup of grated Parmesan cheese
- Cooking spray

Preheat your oven to 350 degrees and prepare a baking sheet. Season each breast with salt and pepper. Next, mix together the basil, garlic, oil and lemon juice. Put each breast in the mixture for five minutes on each side. Mix together the cheese and breadcrumbs on a small plate and coat each breast. Finally, bake for thirty minutes and then serve.

**Fish Cakes**

You will need:

- Two baking potatoes
- One can of white beans, drained
- Half a cup of tartar sauce
- One quarter cup of yeast
- One small spoon of powdered kelp
- One small spoon of spicy paprika
- A dash of salt
- A dash of pepper
- Three cups of grated zucchini
- One cup of gluten-free flour
- Oil

Peel each potato and cut into smaller pieces. Boil in a pan filled with salt water for fifteen minutes. Rinse and then place in a food processor, along with the tartar sauce, kelp, paprika, salt, pepper and yeast. Pulse together until smooth. Stir the zucchini into the mixture and then add half a cup of the flour. Over a medium flame, heat up the oil. Break the mixture into eight balls and then roll them in the remaining flour. Flatten each one into a cake shape. Cook each patty in the pan for five minutes on each side.

**Squash Pasta**

You will need:

- One butternut squash, peeled and chopped
- A dash of salt
- A dash of pepper
- Eight ounces of gluten-free penne
- One small spoon of nutmeg
- One small spoon of rosemary
- One grated garlic clove
- One quarter cup of Parmesan cheese
- A handful of chopped walnuts
- A handful of chopped dried cranberries

Put the chopped squash in a pan with an inch of water and a dash of salt. Allow it to start boiling and then let it go for fifteen minutes. While you wait, boil another large pot of salt water and cook the penne. Set aside two cups of water from the pasta and drain it. When the squash is done, drain it and mash it up before returning it to the pan. Add in the garlic, nutmeg and rosemary. Cook for about five minutes over low heat. Slowly add in the cheese. Next, add in the squash along with a cup of the pasta water. Mix together until it becomes creamy. Top off with salt, pepper, walnuts and cranberries.

## Corn Chowder Soup

You will need:

- One large spoon of butter, unsalted
- One piece of bacon
- One half cup of chopped onion
- One third cup of chopped carrot
- One third cup of chopped celery
- Two cups of corn kernels, cobs reserved
- One bay leaf
- Three and a half cups of milk
- One peeled and diced Russet potato
- One quarter cup of chopped red bell pepper
- Salt and pepper
- Half a small spoon of thyme leaves

Over medium heat, melt the butter in a large pan. Add in the bacon and fry for four minutes only. Next, add the onion and sauté it for five minutes. Add in the carrot and celery and cook for another five. Break each corn cob in half and add to the mixture. Next, put in the bay leaf and milk. Allow it all to boil and then reduce heat and simmer while covered. Let it cook for a half hour. After that, take out the cobs, bacon and bay leaf. Return the heat to medium and add in the red pepper, potato, salt and pepper. Simmer again for fifteen minutes. Again, return the heat to medium and add the thyme and corn kernels. Allow it to boil and then simmer for another five minutes before serving.

## Gluten-Free Cilantro Tacos

You will need:

- Three large spoons of milk
- Six egg whites
- Two eggs
- One chopped red onion
- One quarter cup of chopped tomato
- One half cup of chopped cilantro
- One large spoon of olive oil, extra-virgin
- One small spoon of ground cumin

- One quarter small spoon of salt
- One can of chopped green chilies
- One cup of cooked brown rice
- Eight gluten-free corn tortillas
- Four wedges of lime

Combine the milk, egg whites, and eggs and whisk together. In a separate bowl, combine the onion, tomato, cilantro, olive oil, ground cumin, salt and chilies and stir. Slowly add in the rice while stirring. Cover it and keep it warm. Over medium heat, coat a skillet with cooking spray and add the egg mixture. Cook for two minutes and stir when it begins to set. Draw a spatula throw it to form curds. Cook until it thickens. Remove from stove top and warm up the corn tortillas. Spoon the egg mixture into the tortillas followed by the rice mixture. Fold in half to form a taco and then serve with lime.

## Cajun Catfish

You will need:

- Four 6oz catfish fillets
- A small amount of Cajun seasoning
- One dash of salt
- Half a cup of mayonnaise
- One large spoon of sweet relish
- One large spoon of minced onion
- One large spoon of drained capers
- One small spoon of hot sauce
- A small amount of dried oregano

Over medium heat, coat a skillet with cooking spray and season the catfish with the Cajun seasoning and salt. Cook each fillet for four minutes on each side. As each fillet cooks, you can combine the mayonnaise, relish, onion, capers, hot sauce and oregano and serve it up as a side to the fish.

## Indian Style Salmon

You will need:

- One small spoon of ground ginger
- Half a small spoon of garam masala
- Half a small spoon of ground coriander
- One small spoon of ground turmeric
- Kosher salt
- Ground red pepper
- Four 6oz salmon fillets

Preheat your broiler and cover a baking pan with cooking spray. Place the salmon fillets in the pan and combine the other ingredients together, evenly spreading the mixture out on the fillets. Cover with aluminum foil and cook for seven minutes. Remove the foil and and then broil for another four minutes. Serve when done.

**Merlot-Balsamic Sirloin Steak**

You will need:

- Half a cup of Merlot
- Two large spoons of balsamic vinegar
- One large spoon of gluten-free Worcestershire sauce
- Half a small spoon of ground pepper
- One dash of salt
- One pound of sirloin steak, boneless and trimmed
- One large spoon of canola oil
- Half a cup of chopped shallots

In a big Ziploc bag, combine the merlot, balsamic vinegar, Worcestershire sauce, ground pepper and salt. Put the steak in the bag next and marinate for 15 minutes, being sure to completely coat the steak. Over medium heat, spray a skillet with cooking spray and transfer the steak from the bag to the pan. Cook for five minutes on each side and then lower heat and cook for another three minutes on each side. Set the steak aside. Next, add the oil to the pan and cook the shallots for two minutes. Stir in the remaining marinade from the bag and bring to a boil for two minutes. Cut the steak into thin strips and spoon the new sauce over it to serve.

**Gluten-Free Chicken Fried Steak**

You will need:

- One cup of breading mix
- Two cups of soy milk
- Two eggs
- Four 4oz cubed steaks
- Two large spoons of canola oil
- One large spoon of corn starch
- Half a small spoon of salt
- Half a small spoon of pepper
- Four small spoons of chopped parsley

In a bowl, pour in the breading mix. In another bowl, mix half a cup of soy milk and the eggs. Stir together with a whisk. Dip each steak in the breading and then cover each with the egg mixture. Cover a skillet with cooking spray and heat one large spoon of oil over medium heat. Fry two steaks at a time for four minutes on each side. In a measuring cup, combine the remaining milk, cornstarch, salt and pepper. Stir this mixture into the leftover drippings in the pan used to cook the steaks. Boil over medium to high heat and cook for one minute, stirring occasionally. Spoon this over the steaks and then top with the chopped parsley.

**Smokey Pork Tenderloin**

You will need:

- One large spoon of brown sugar
- One and a half small spoons of smoked paprika
- One small spoon of garlic powder
- One small spoon of espresso granules
- Half a small spoon of salt
- Half a small spoon of onion powder
- Half a small spoon of ground pepper
- One pound of trimmed pork tenderloin
- One small spoon of olive oil
- Half a cup of water

Preheat your oven to 425 degrees and combine the sugar, paprika, garlic powder, granules, salt, onion powder, and ground pepper in a bowl. Spread the mixture on the tenderloin and let sit for 20 minutes. Over medium to high heat, cover a skillet with cooking spray and heat the oil. Cook the tenderloin for two minutes on each side then bake for 20 minutes. Remove the tenderloin from the oven and cover for 10 minutes. Stir in the water to the leftover drippings and then spread that sauce over the pork to serve.

**Spicy Grilled Chicken**

You will need:

- One small spoon of onion powder
- One small spoon of garlic powder
- One small spoon of dried oregano
- Half a small spoon of salt
- Half a small spoon of cayenne pepper
- Half a small spoon of black pepper
- Four 6oz chicken breasts

Preheat your grill to medium-high. In a bowl, combine the spices together and spread over each chicken breast evenly. Spray the grill rack with cooking spray and grill each breast for six minutes on each side. If you enjoy the spice rub, you can additionally keep it ready-made, stored in an airtight container for future use.

**Mango-Avocado Chicken Tacos**

You will need:

- One small spoon of garlic powder
- One dash of paprika
- One small spoon of onion powder
- One dash of red pepper
- One dash of salt
- Four 6oz chicken breasts
- One large spoon of olive oil
- Half a cup of peeled mango, diced
- Half a cup of peeled avocado, diced
- Half a cup of tomato, chopped
- A handful of chopped cilantro
- Two large spoons of lime juice
- One large spoon of jalapeno pepper, minced
- Four gluten-free brown rice tortillas

In a bowl, add together the garlic powder, paprika, onion powder, and red pepper in a skillet while adding in a dash of salt. Spread it on each chicken breast and then add the oil to a skillet over medium-high heat. Cook the chicken for four minutes on each side. Once done, cut each chicken breast into thin slices. As the chicken is cooking, get another bowl and mix together the mango, avocado, chopped tomatoes, chopped cilantro, lime juice and jalapeno pepper. Once that is mixed together, add in another quarter small spoon of salt. Heat up the tortillas and then fill with the chicken and salsa mixture.

# Conclusion

I hope this book was able to help you to learn more about Gluten, Gluten Intolerance, Celiac disease and a healthier diet. I would highly recommend keeping a food journal for a month and writing down all the changes you made to your diet, the foods you eat each day and your overall wellbeing and energy levels for each day. If you can determine the optimum diet for yourself, you are one giant step closer to living at your full potential! Remember, while you may not even suffer from Celiac disease, maintaining a gluten-free diet can still have its benefits, mostly due to the overall higher quality of the foods that you'd eat.

The next step is to try out some of the recipes! Start out by experimenting with some of the snacks for yourself. Once you've gotten really good at making these dishes, feel free to search through the others and make the ones that most appeal to you. Once you have found your favorites, enjoy them again and again, knowing that they are delicious and full of energy! I hope both you and/or your family are able to enjoy the dishes listed throughout this book. Be creative and see what you can come up with from here—you don't necessarily have to stick to the same recipe or ingredients each time. Everyone is different, so find out what works best for you or the ones you love!

Finally, if you discovered at least one thing that has helped you or that you think would be beneficial to someone else, be sure to take a few seconds to easily post a quick positive review. As an author, your positive feedback is desperately needed. Your highly valuable five star reviews are like a river of golden joy flowing through a sunny forest of mighty trees and beautiful flowers! *To do your good deed in making the world a better place by helping others with your valuable insight, just leave a nice review.*

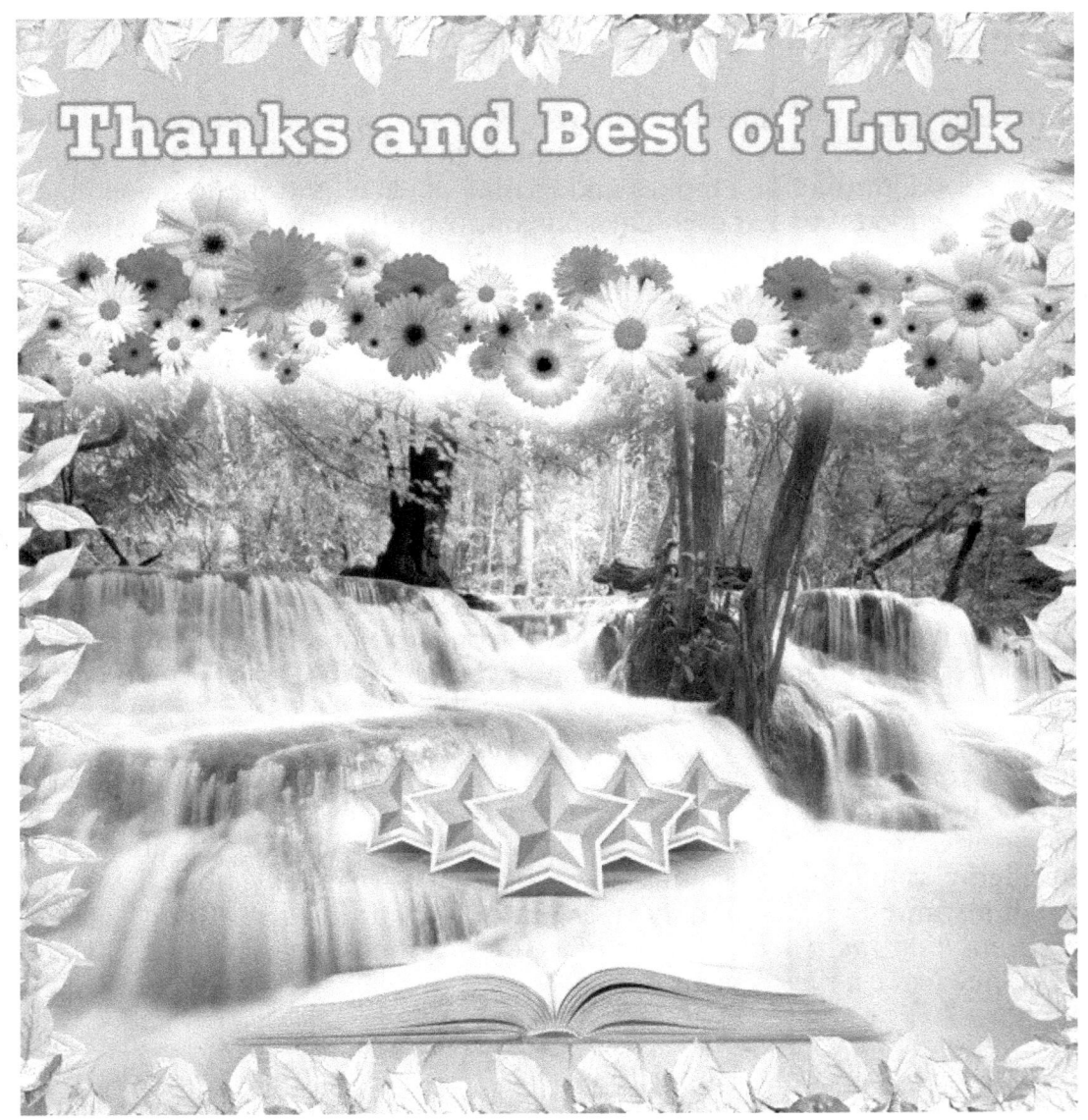

**My Other Books and Audio Books**
www.AcesEbooks.com

# Health Books

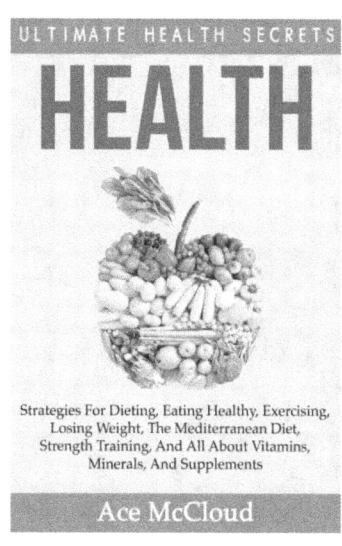
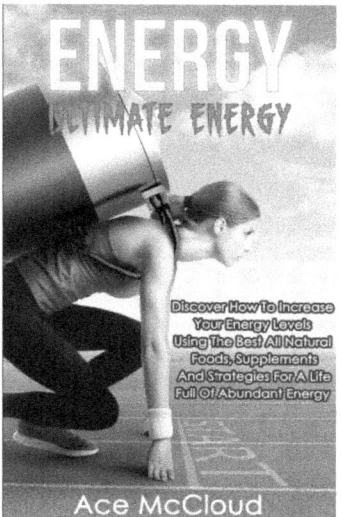
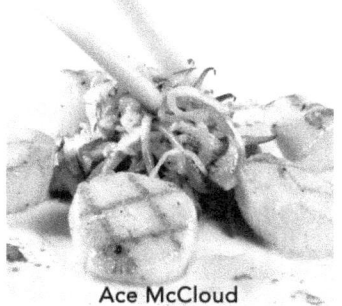
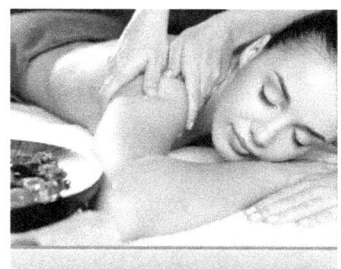
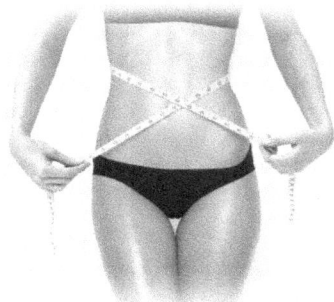
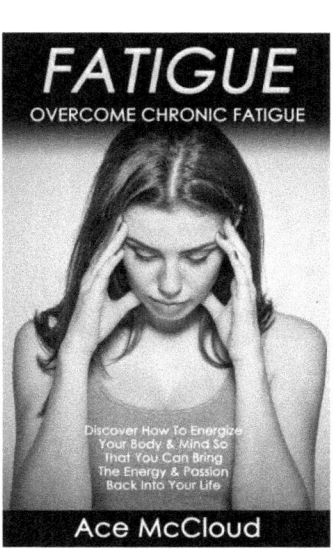

# Peak Performance Books

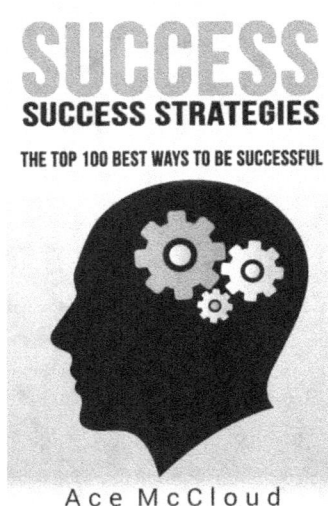
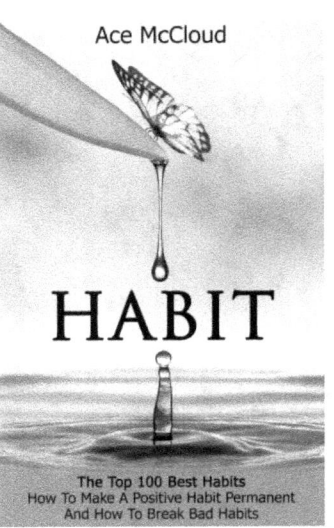
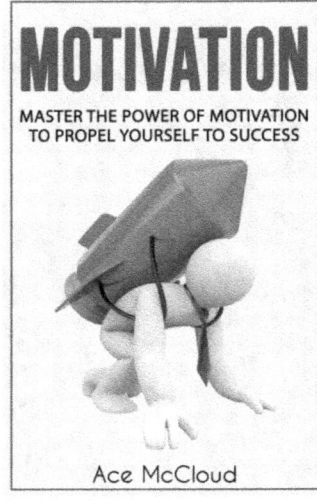
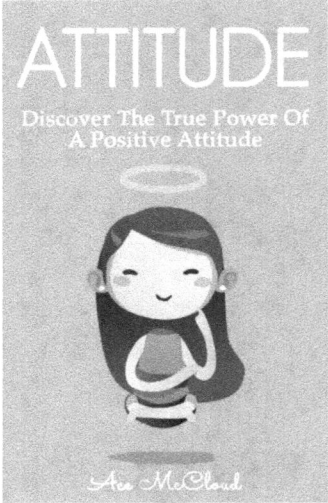

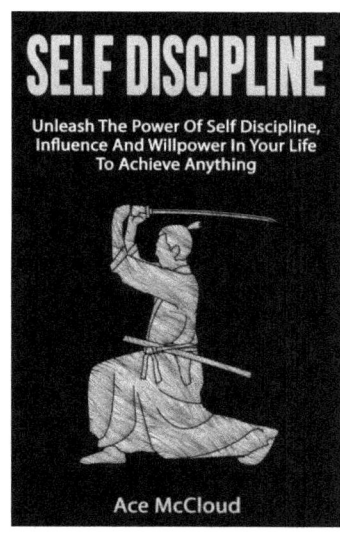 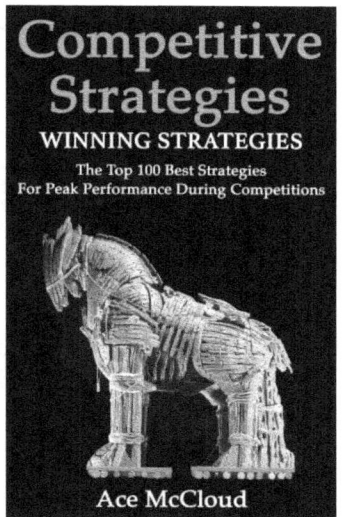

# Be sure to check out my audio books as well!

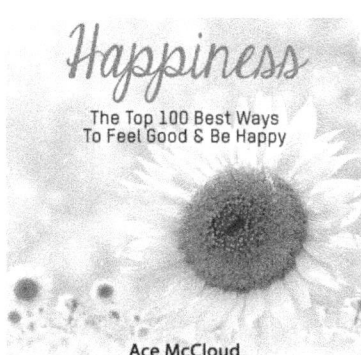 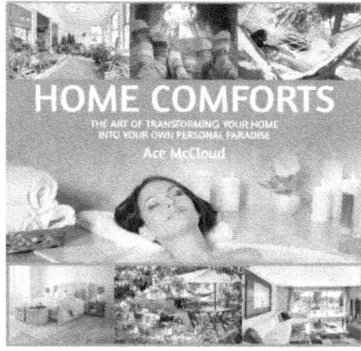 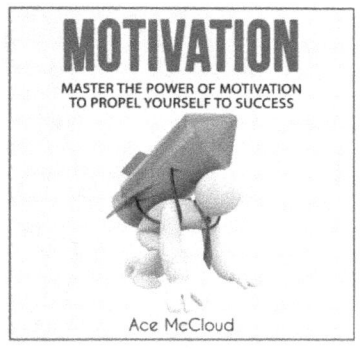

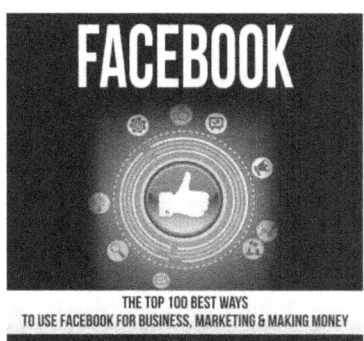 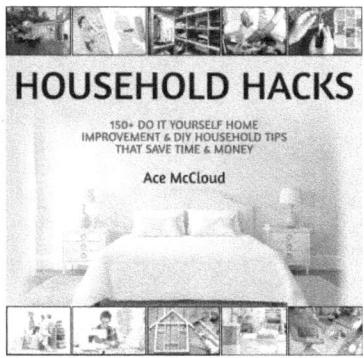 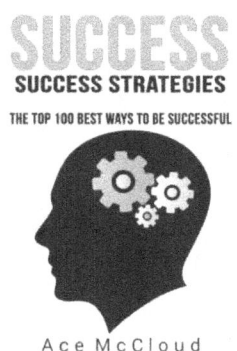

Check out my website at: **www.AcesEbooks.com** for a complete list of all of my books and high quality audio books. I enjoy bringing you the best knowledge in the world and wish you the best in using this information to make your journey through life better and more enjoyable! **Best of luck to you!**

www.ingramcontent.com/pod-product-compliance
Lightning Source LLC
Chambersburg PA
CBHW051426070526
44584CB00023B/3606